10 Benefits of Maintaining a Healthy Lifestyle

Healthy Lifestyle

ABDULKADIR MANYA TAFIDA

ii

DEDICATION

This book is dedicated to my Wife, Mrs. Salamatu Umar, my daughter and to the whole of my family.

CONTENTS

INTRODUCTION

There are so many benefits to maintaining a healthy lifestyle! Your body will be able to do so much more if it's healthy, and if you maintain a healthy lifestyle, you can prevent so many illnesses and diseases that could potentially shorten your life and reduce your quality of life. There are 10 benefits of maintaining a healthy lifestyle, and I think they're all really important!

BOOSTS ENERGY LEVELS

A healthy diet boosts your energy levels and can provide you with more stamina to get through your day. Eating smaller, more frequent meals throughout the day is beneficial for maintaining steady blood sugar levels, which in turn helps promote better sleep and mood regulation. If you're feeling sluggish or low on energy, try eating some protein-rich foods and vegetables. Protein will keep your blood sugar levels stable and help build muscle mass, which can lead to an increase in energy.

REDUCES THE RISK OF CHRONIC DISEASES

A healthy lifestyle can reduce the risk of chronic diseases and help prevent new ones from forming. For example, studies have shown that those who maintain a healthy weight are less likely to develop diabetes or heart disease. This is because being overweight puts excess stress on your body and increases your risk for developing insulin resistance. In addition, eating too much junk food can lead to an increased risk for diseases such as cancer or pancreatitis. It's important not just to focus on what you eat but also how much you eat because overeating can cause many issues with your liver, pancreas, and digestive system. A healthy lifestyle will also help you avoid problems such as high blood pressure and cardiovascular disease which can lead to stroke or heart attack.

Lifestyle and health-related behaviours are powerful determinants of morbidity and mortality worldwide, and unhealthy behaviours lie at the root of many chronic and disabling diseases. Major concerns focus on smoking, body mass, physical activity, diet and alcohol consumption, and the concept of a healthy lifestyle is usually defined with reference to combinations of these factors. A number of studies have shown that the following of lifestyles based on these factors is strongly associated with reductions in the incidence of certain chronic diseases. Indeed, as one writer put it: 'Healthy living is the best revenge.

Lifestyles, and in particular physical activity have been shown to be associated with cognitive health. Several reviews however have commented that the quality of the evidence is low and have called for more long-term cohort studies before conclusions can be drawn with confidence about the role of healthy behaviours in cognitive health. A major issue is reverse causation. While this is a concern with all the outcomes, it is an especial concern in relation to dementia, because the pathophysiological processes associated with Alzheimer's Disease are known to begin many years prior to detectable cognitive impairment. Evidence from short-term studies is therefore limited, seriously in the case of cognitive impairment, and long-term studies are greatly to be preferred.

The personal and public health benefits from healthy behaviours have been shown to have enormous potential so it is important that the uptake is carefully monitored. Evidence from a number of studies in the UK [4] [7] and elsewhere [6] [17] [5] show that the uptake of truly healthy lifestyles is very poor.

The Caerphilly Prospective Study (CaPS) is based on a cohort of men in a typical small town in South Wales UK. The men have been repeatedly questioned and examined for over 30 years. In this report we summarise evidence on relationships between healthy lifestyles at baseline and the incidence of diabetes, vascular disease, cancer, all-cause mortality, cognitive impairment and dementia during follow-up. We also examine changes in the following of healthy behaviours over the thirty years.

IMPROVES MENTAL HEALTH

Living a healthy lifestyle isn't always easy, especially during these unique times. Remember, small changes are all you need. Gradually making small changes – like going for a walk, doing an exercise snack or choosing healthier options – can go a long way to ensuring that you focus on regularly adding exercise to your life.

Studies have shown that people with healthy lifestyles experience improved mental health. Exercise, for example, releases endorphins which can help reduce depression and anxiety. Stress is also reduced by maintaining healthy habits such as eating well and getting enough sleep. In the long run, this could lead to lower rates of depression or anxiety disorders.

Your mental health influences how you think, feel, and behave in daily life. It also affects your ability to cope with stress, overcome challenges, build relationships, and recover from life's setbacks and hardships. Strong mental health isn't just the absence of mental health problems. Being mentally or emotionally healthy is much more than being free of depression, anxiety, or other psychological issues. Rather than the absence of mental illness, mental health refers to the presence of positive characteristics.

Getting the recommended amount of exercise can also lead to beneficial changes in mood, anxiety and depression.

Exercise improves mental health by reducing anxiety, stress, depression and negative mood, and by improving cognitive function. Muscle-strengthening activities should be included in an exercise routine, twice a week. This includes yoga, strength training with free weights, resistance band exercises and bodyweight exercises such as pushups, lunges and squats. Aerobic exercises, such as walking, gardening, swimming, running and cycling, have been shown to reduce anxiety and depression. One to two hours of exercise per week have been shown to reduce the risk of depression.

INCREASES LIFE EXPECTANCY

A healthy lifestyle may allow older people to live longer, with women adding three years and men six to their life expectancy, suggests research published in the journal BMJ. In addition, more of those years may be dementia-free. More than 6 million Americans 65 and older have the most common type of dementia, Alzheimer's, for which there is no cure.

The study found that, at age 65, women with the healthiest lifestyle had an average life expectancy of about 24 years, compared with 21 years for women whose lifestyle was deemed less healthy. Life expectancy for men with the healthiest lifestyle was 23 years, vs. 17 years for men who were less healthy.

There are many benefits to maintaining a healthy lifestyle. One benefit is that by leading a healthier life, you will increase your life expectancy. The Centers for Disease Control and Prevention found that poor lifestyle habits have accounted for 25% of all deaths in the United States from 2000-2014. By making small changes in your daily habits, you can significantly improve your health and reduce those risks.

a) Increases Life Expectancy

b) Decreases Stress

c) Reduces Pain

d) Increases Energy Levels

e) Improves Self-Esteem

f) Improves Sleep Quality

g) Decreases Risks of Certain Cancers

REDUCES HEALTHCARE COSTS

Studies show that maintaining a healthy lifestyle can reduce your healthcare costs by up to 40%. Reducing your healthcare costs can help you save money, spend less time at the doctor's office, and stay out of the hospital. Don't let medical expenses derail you from living life to the fullest. Start taking care of yourself and reap these benefits.

Health and wealth are related in many different ways. First, there is the sheer cost of unhealthy habits. Eliminate a $10 a day smoking or junk food habit, for example, and you can save $3,650 annually, plus interest. That's just the immediate savings. There are also savings over the long term for the rest of someone's life. The Centers for Disease Control estimates that a 10% weight loss could reduce an overweight person's lifetime medical costs by $2,200 to $5,300. Delaying the onset of diabetes can save thousands of dollars annually in increased medical costs.

Secondly, financial problems can affect a person's health status and vice versa. For example, overdue medical bills can result in physical symptoms of stress (e.g., migraines, insomnia, and anxiety) and/or delayed or inadequate treatment. Financial distress also makes it difficult to afford recommended health maintenance practices, such as routine check-ups and eating the recommended 5 to 9 servings of fruits and vegetables per day. High health costs can lead to a poor credit history and/or bankruptcy and reduced income available to save for retirement and other financial goals. Medical problems were found to be associated with about half the cases of bankruptcy filed in 2001.

A third health and wealth relationship is that people in poor health often die at a relatively young age and spend thousands of dollars--money that could otherwise have been invested—on prescription drugs and health care costs. Many don't live long enough to collect the pension and Social Security benefits that they spent a lifetime working for. On the other hand, those who practice recommended health behaviors will more likely exceed average life expectancy and need a large retirement nest egg to insure that they don't outlive their assets. Most financial planners routinely plan for life expectancies in the mid 90s to assure that their clients don't run out of money.

PREVENTS OBESITY

Obesity is an illness that is associated with excess body weight. It is a step ahead of being overweight. Obesity can trigger a lot of other problems in the human body. It makes you vulnerable to diabetes, heart issues, and life-threatening diseases such as cancer.

Multiple factors are responsible for making a person obese. Family history, sedentary lifestyle, and lack of a balanced diet are major causes of obesity. Knowing your Body Mass Index (BMI) is a good way to understand whether you fall under the following categories – underweight, normal, overweight, and obese. You can speak with a medical professional to know your BMI accurately.

A healthy lifestyle has many benefits, including preventing obesity. According to the Centers for Disease Control and Prevention (CDC), 1 in 3 adults in the United States are obese. Obesity is caused by over-consuming calories and not burning enough calories through exercise. A healthy lifestyle can prevent obesity as it decreases your risk for diabetes, high blood pressure, heart disease, stroke, and cancer. Additionally, maintaining a healthy weight will also allow you to feel more energized and confident. If you need some ideas on how to live a healthier life, take a look at our list below.

Obesity can be prevented, provided you lead a disciplined life. For example, if you are overweight, then controlling your diet and exercising can prevent you from becoming obese. It can also reduce your weight. Listed below are five weight-management tips that can help you to prevent obesity.

1. Eat the Right Stuff:

A balanced diet constitutes healthy food items that provide your body with adequate nutrients. Food items that have a high proportion of salt and sugar are dangerous for the body. Avoid binging on fast-food, drinking excessive alcohol, and smoking. Consuming fried stuff on a regular basis is also a big no. People tend to overeat if there's a huge gap between two meals. Avoid that. Eat healthy food items at frequent intervals. Pampering your taste buds with pizzas and pastries is fine if it is done occasionally.

2. Exercise, it Feels Good!:

Exercising shouldn't be a task. It should be a fun activity; something that you look forward to. A lot of people have the misconception that exercising means lifting heavy weights and sweating it out in the gym. That is just one aspect of exercising, not the only one. There are multiple ways in which you can ensure that you are involved in some kind of physical activity. Swimming, dancing, jogging, etc. are also ways to burn extra calories and workout your muscles.

3. Sleeping has More to Offer:

People usually associate sleeping with getting rest. A sound sleep does more than that for your body and mind. It influences neuroendocrine cells, glucose metabolism, and other functions that are responsible for enabling smooth bodily functions. For example, lack of sleep can harm appetite-related hormones, which can lead to excess eating resulting in obesity.

4. Stay Consistent:

Regularity is of great essence in managing body weight. Eating right, exercising right, and sleeping right needs regularity. Doing so for a month and then going off-schedule for the next isn't going to help the cause. Monitor the above-mentioned activities and take active measures if you are going off-track.

5. Beat the Stress:

Stress can mess with your mind and body in multiple ways. If you find yourself in a situation where you are fatigued and sleep-deprived for a long period of time, it is time to take control of your life and control the stress-causing factors. Crumbling under stress can cause metabolic imbalances leading to a host of problems, including obesity. Visit your doctor at the earliest and take corrective measures in case you feel stressed out on a continuous basis.

REDUCES STRESS LEVELS

Walking, exercising, and eating healthier foods are all ways to reduce your stress levels. Exercise increases the production of endorphins in your body which makes you feel happy and relaxed. It also helps release chemicals that make you feel good like serotonin and dopamine. Walking is a great way to exercise because it doesn't require any equipment or special skills. It's simple, free, and can be done anywhere! Adding fruits, vegetables, whole grains, or protein sources to your diet will help control cravings for sugar or carbs. Proper nutrition will also keep you full which can help prevent overeating and weight gain. Eating healthy not only reduces stress levels but it also reduces the risk of developing chronic diseases such as diabetes or heart disease.

IMPROVES SKIN COMPLEXION

A healthy lifestyle can improve your skin complexion by reducing inflammation and drying out your skin, which will result in fewer wrinkles. It also helps to maintain collagen production that keeps your skin firm and elastic. If you have acne-prone skin, healthy habits can help reduce breakouts and prevent clogged pores. Your hair will also benefit from healthy habits as it promotes growth for healthier locks. Plus, a healthy lifestyle will help you sleep better at night, reduce anxiety and depression levels, as well as increase energy levels.

While we can't stop the natural aging process, our lifestyle choices can play a significant role in maintaining healthy, glowing skin. Avoiding excess sun exposure, wearing sunscreen, drinking less alcohol and not smoking are the most crucial steps to take in protecting and healing your skin. Healthy habits like getting regular exercise and staying hydrated can also help promote a beautiful glowing complexion in addition to overall health and wellness. But one of the most satisfying ways to slow premature aging is to eat delicious foods full of nutrients that work together to support and maintain the daily functions of the skin.

A general rule of thumb when it comes to understanding the best foods for healthy skin is to shift towards eating more of a Mediterranean-style diet. Known for its emphasis on antioxidant-rich foods, a Mediterranean diet includes a variety of beneficial nutrients that can function as bodyguards to skin cells and protect them from damage. Foods packed with water, like the fruits and vegetables abundant in a Mediterranean diet, can help hydrate the skin. Probiotic-rich ones like Greek yogurt can provide beneficial bacteria to support a healthy gut, which is vital to maintaining healthy skin.

With that in mind, here are the best foods to eat for healthy skin at any age, according to registered dietitians:

1. Bell Peppers

Not only are they delicious, but bell peppers are one of the best vitamin C-rich foods and pack in 95mg — over 100% of the daily value for vitamin C — in just half a cup. Vitamin C has important antioxidant properties and is known for its immune-supporting benefits, but it plays a significant role in skin health too.

Vitamin C can prevent and treat skin damage from ultraviolet (UV) light and even plays a role in wound healing. The antioxidant is also important for collagen synthesis. We know that many environmental pollutants can decrease vitamin C levels in the skin and lead to free radical damage, so incorporating vitamin C-rich foods into the diet is key.

Add sliced peppers to salads and sandwiches or transform them into delicious red pepper hummus for a yummy way to reap the benefits of this favorite vegetable.

2. Watermelon

Every single cell in your body needs water to function properly and optimally, which is why foods with a high-water content are helpful for meeting your daily hydration needs. Two cups of cubed watermelon equal a full cup of water and can help you (and therefore your skin cells) stay hydrated and maintain skin elasticity.

But that isn't the only thing going for this delicious fruit. The beta-carotene and vitamin C found in watermelon makes it an antioxidant-packed snack that can help fight inflammation and free radicals in the skin.

Try cutting it up and storing it in the freezer for a treat during warmer months. You can even transform it into a festive watermelon pizza or enjoy it with a savorier twist in a delightful watermelon feta salad.

INCREASES PRODUCTIVITY

Are all these extra hours and minimum days off proving to be more productive for businesses? In the long run, the short answer is no. The real issue is the detrimental impact this kind of poor work-life balance is having on workers. There is actually a scientific link between work-life balance, employee engagement and productivity – a more balanced work-lifestyle can lead to higher productivity.

According to a study by the Corporate Leadership Council, people who feel they have good work-life balance work 21% harder than those who don't. Workers who feel they have some flexibility in how they do their tasks and take care of their home and life responsibilities respond in a proactive way that encourages them to engage and do more. In the academic world, this is termed the Social Exchange Theory. An employer or organization offers benefits or incentives to the employee, and the employee reciprocates in the form of going above and beyond the call of duty.

Contrastingly, studies have found the negative effects of poor work-life balance can lead to reduced work effort and performance. It can also lead to increased absenteeism and turnover, reduced health and energy, and increased stress.

Maintaining a healthy lifestyle can improve your productivity. Here are some benefits to consider:

(a) Better sleep;

(b) Increased mental clarity and creativity;

(c) Greater energy levels;

(d) Improved concentration, focus, and attention span;

(e) Reduced risk of illness due to better immune function;

(f) Weight loss and improved muscle tone.

ABOUT THE AUTHOR

Abdulkadir Manya Tafida is a Bachelor's Degree holder in Biological Science and currently running his MSc program in Environmental Biology as at when writing this book.